DYSPNEA

FEW WAYS OUT OF DYSPNEA

DR. J. SIMON

Contents

INTRODUCTION

Dyspnea is a subjective experience of difficulty or discomfort in breathing. It is sometimes referred to as shortness of breath or breathlessness. It is a symptom, not a particular medical ailment, and it can be brought on by a number of underlying disorders that damage the body's circulatory, respiratory, or other systems.

People who experience dyspnea may describe feeling as though they are not getting enough oxygen, that their chest feels constricted, or that their breathing is happening too quickly. Dyspnea can be modest and temporary, as it happens after intensive physical exertion, or severe and chronic, demanding medical attention.

There are various different conditions that can cause dyspnea, including interstitial lung disease, pneumonia, asthma, and chronic obstructive pulmonary disease (COPD). Breathlessness may also be caused by cardiovascular disorders such as coronary artery disease, arrhythmias, or heart failure. Non-respiratory factors may also be involved, including anxiety, obesity, anemia, and neuromuscular disorders.

Finding and addressing the underlying cause of dyspnea is an important element of its assessment and treatment. Healthcare experts may undertake diagnostic testing, such as pulmonary function tests, imaging investigations, or blood tests, to discover the underlying cause, dependant on the strength and type of the illness.

Dyspnea has a number of explanations, so a complete evaluation is important to establish the best course of treatment. Depending on the underlying condition, management techniques may comprise medication, lifestyle adjustments, pulmonary rehabilitation, or surgical interventions.

Dyspnea can influence a person's everyday activities and quality of life, which underlines the necessity of timely and comprehensive medical evaluation. Seeking prompt medical aid is vital for an accurate diagnosis and proper therapy if someone is experiencing severe or chronic dyspnea.

CHAPTER ONE

The meaning of dyspnea

Shortness of breath, or dyspnea, is a subjective feeling that is marked by difficulty or discomfort in breathing. Breathlessness, chest tightness, or an increased effort to breathe are all indications of the sense of insufficient or unpleasant breathing.

Dyspnea is a symptom that can be linked to a number of underlying medical diseases that damage the circulatory, respiratory, or other systems; it is not a distinct disease. It can happen for a variety of reasons, from physical strain or anxiety to more serious medical conditions including heart or lung problems.

Dyspnea is a subjective condition that affects various persons differently. People who experience dyspnea might characterize it in a variety of ways, including feeling as though they are not breathing deeply enough, breathing quickly or shallowly, or experiencing tightness in their chest.

A full medical evaluation, which includes a review of medical history, physical examination, and maybe additional diagnostic testing such pulmonary function tests, imaging studies, or blood tests, is often essential to identify and diagnose the cause of dyspnea.

Finding and addressing the underlying cause is key to controlling dyspnea. Medication, lifestyle changes, pulmonary rehabilitation, or procedures particular to the specified disease are among viable therapy options.

Dyspnea can have a major affect on a person's daily activities and general well-being. Therefore, it is vital to seek medical assistance for persistent or severe symptoms in order to acquire an accurate diagnosis and adequate care.

The Value of Diagnosing and Treating Dyspnea

Dyspnea, or shortness of breath, must be detected and treated for a number of essential reasons.

A symptom of underlying medical conditions

Dyspnea typically suggests the existence of an underlying medical problem, which can include heart failure or coronary artery disease as well as respiratory diseases like asthma or chronic obstructive pulmonary disease (COPD). Early dyspnea discovery can help with these underlying disorders' diagnosis and treatment.

Impact on Quality of Life:

Dyspnea has a huge effect on a person's quality of life. It might make it more difficult for individuals to go about their normal lives, work exercise, or participate in social and leisure activities. By addressing dyspnea, people can live more active and satisfying lives and experience an overall improvement in their general well-being.

Early Serious Condition Identification:

Dyspnea can occasionally be an indication of serious conditions that could be fatal, like abrupt heart failure or pulmonary embolism. Accurate identification and quick medical intervention may be necessary to addressing these situations successfully.

Handling Prolonged Illnesses:

Early dyspnea detection offers improved treatment and control of long-term respiratory or cardiovascular diseases in affected patients. Complications and exacerbations can be avoided with the correct therapy and lifestyle adjustments.

Impact on the Mind:

Anxiety and anguish are associated to dyspnea. People who are having breathing problems may become afraid or nervous about their breathing. Treating dyspnea has a substantial impact on mental and emotional health in addition to physical health.

Tailored Care Programs:

The ability to define the precise cause of dyspnea allows medical providers to build individualized therapy regimens. Different therapies are needed for different conditions, and identifying dyspnea permits focused interventions to address the underlying cause.

Preventive actions:

Early diagnosis affords the possibility to take preventive action when dyspnea is linked to lifestyle factors like obesity or sedentary behavior. Making lifestyle adjustments like controlling your weight and exercising frequently can help lessen your probability of having respiratory and cardiovascular disorders or making them worse.

Enhanced Results for Patients:

Better patient outcomes are a result of dyspnea being detected and treated immediately. Prompt identification and action can arrest the advancement of certain disorders, minimize complications, and enhance general health results.

People who have severe or chronic dyspnea should contact a doctor since dyspnea can be caused by a wide range of disorders. Appropriate steps can be initiated by this awareness and the accompanying medical evaluation, enhancing health and well-being.

The Physiology and Anatomy of Breathing

Dyspnea can be induced by abnormalities in the complicated connections between the respiratory and cardiovascular systems, which are crucial to the architecture and physiology of breathing. Knowing the foundations of breathing highlights the probable reasons of dyspnea:

1. The respiratory system

Lungs: The respiratory system's main organs, the lungs, contribute in the exchange of carbon dioxide and oxygen. During breath, oxygen is taken in, and during expiration, carbon dioxide is exhaled.

The airways that branch from the trachea and travel into the lungs are referred to as bronchi and bronchioles. These further split into smaller bronchioles, which eventually create alveoli, which are air sacs.

Alveoli: The locations of gas exchange are these tiny, thin-walled sacs. While blood's carbon dioxide travels into the alveoli to be evacuated during expiration, oxygen from the breathing air diffuses into the bloodstream.

2. Muscles Used for Inhalation:

The diaphragm is a muscular dome that divides the chambers of the chest and abdomen. Air can enter the lungs during inhalation because the diaphragm contracts, increasing the thoracic cavity.

Intercostal Muscles: These muscles help to expand and compress the chest while breathing. They are positioned between the ribs.

3. Breathing Control via the Nerves:

Breathing is regulated by the brain's respiratory center, which is contained in the medulla oblongata and pons. It reacts to fluctuations in the blood's pH, oxygen, and carbon dioxide contents.

Respiratory muscles contract in response to brain signals, which modify the depth and speed of breathing.

4. Heart System:

Heart: The heart takes in deoxygenated blood from the body and pumps oxygenated blood to the tissues. Together with the respiratory system, the cardiovascular system makes sure that the body obtains enough oxygen to meet its demands.

Blood Circulation: The left atrium of the heart receives oxygenated blood from the lungs, which is subsequently pumped into the systemic circulation. Blood that has lost oxygen is returned to the right atrium of the heart and is sent to the lungs to pick up oxygen.

Dyspnea

When the body's need for oxygen is greater than what the respiratory and cardiovascular systems can deliver, dyspnea may develop.

Dyspnea may be brought on by cardiovascular diseases (heart failure, pulmonary embolism), respiratory ailments (asthma, COPD), or other conditions (obesity, anxiety).

When someone has dyspnea, their breathing rate or effort may increase due to signals given to the respiratory center of the brain suggesting that they need more oxygen or that the oxygen supply is not sufficient.

Breathing-related muscles may become weak or exhausted, which can increase the impression of problems breathing.

An study of the anatomy and physiology of breathing is important to appreciate how pauses in these complicated systems can produce dyspnea. Addressing the underlying abnormalities effecting respiratory and cardiovascular function is often part of the treatment and management of dyspnea.

Reasons for Dyspnea

A multitude of disorders affecting the respiratory, cardiovascular, or other systems of the body can result in dyspnea, or shortness of breath. Determining the core issue is key to efficient management. Following are a few typical causes of dyspnea:

Conditions Related to the Respiratory System:

Chronic airway inflammation that causes bronchoconstriction and breathing difficulties is known as asthma.

A collection of progressive lung disorders typified by airflow obstruction, including emphysema and chronic bronchitis, is known as chronic obstructive pulmonary disease, or COPD.

Disorders that hinder oxygen exchange by inflaming and scarring lung tissue are known as interstitial lung disorders.

Pneumonia: Inflammation and infection of the lung tissue that results in air sacs filled with fluid.

Heart-Related Disorders:

Heart Failure: When the heart cannot efficiently pump blood, fluid accumulates in the lungs (pulmonary edema).

A narrowing or blockage of the coronary arteries that reduces blood flow to the heart muscle is known as coronary artery disease (CAD).

Arrhythmias: Abnormal cardiac rhythms that affect the heart's capacity to pump blood.

Blood clots clogging the pulmonary arteries produce pulmonary embolism, which reduces blood flow to the lungs.

Anemia

diminished blood's ability to carry oxygen as a result of a decline in hemoglobin or red blood cells.

Overweight:

Being overweight exerts stress on the heart and lungs, which can induce dyspnea, especially when exercising.

Disorders of Anxiety and Panic:

Breathlessness can be brought on by emotional reasons like anxiety or panic attacks.

Deconditioning

A prolonged period of bed rest or inactivity can harm the muscles of the heart and lungs.

Heart Hypertension:

higher pulmonary artery pressure, which makes the heart work harder to pump blood to the lungs.

GERD, or gastroesophageal reflux disease:

Breathing issues can come from stomach acid reflux affecting the esophagus and aggravating the airways.

Neuromuscular Conditions:

illnesses include amyotrophic lateral sclerosis (ALS) and myasthenia gravis that impair the breathing-related nerves and muscles.

Allergies:

Experiencing severe allergic reactions such as anaphylaxis can lead to bronchoconstriction and trouble breathing.

Injury to the Chest or Trauma:

Dyspnea can be brought on by trauma to the respiratory system or injuries to the chest.

Exposures to the Environment:

Breathing issues may be increased by exposure to air pollution, work-related dangers, or high elevations.

Side effects from medication:

Dyspnea is a side effect of various medicines, especially those that damage the cardiovascular or respiratory systems.

It's crucial to remember that dyspnea is a symptom, not a diagnosis, and that there are many different probable reasons. People who suffer severe or persistent dyspnea should receive medical attention right once for a complete assessment and adequate treatment.

Signs and Suggestions

Dyspnea, sometimes known as shortness of breath, is a subjective condition that causes a person to perceive difficulty or discomfort in breathing. Depending on the underlying reason, dyspnea's signs and symptoms could vary and may include:

Elevated Rate of Respiration:

One of the most common symptoms of dyspnea is fast breathing or a high respiratory rate. The body makes additional breaths in an attempt to make up for what it perceives to be a scarcity of oxygen.

Breathing Too Little:

Breathing may become shallower, with less depth and chest expansion. This can be a reaction to the attempt to alleviate respiratory pain.

Sense of being out of breath:

People who have dyspnea commonly report feeling subjectively breathless, as though they are not breathing deeply enough or are unable to collect enough air.

Constriction in the Chest:

Some patients may feel restricted or restless in their chest, which commonly goes hand in hand with their dyspnea.

Having Trouble Exhaling:

Dyspnea is characterized by problems exhaling, notably in asthmatic or chronic obstructive pulmonary disorders (COPD).

Sighing:

A high-pitched sound that can arise during breathing, especially if the airways are closing, is wheezing. It usually arises in conditions like asthma.

Utilizing Adjacent Muscles:

In extreme cases, people may utilize accessory muscles to aid breathe, such as the muscles in the neck or in between the ribs.

Cyanonoses:

Cyanosis may emerge in instances where dyspnea is connected to low blood oxygen levels. A bluish discoloration of the skin, mainly on the lips and fingertips, is called cyanosis.

Orthopnea:

Orthopnea is the term for difficulties breathing while in a lying position. Some persons with respiratory illnesses or cardiac difficulties may feel better when they sit or stand up straight.

Dyspnea during the night:

Some patients may only suffer dyspnea at night, and they frequently wake up feeling out of breath.

Exercise Intolerance:

Exercise-induced dyspnea is a frequent symptom, particularly in illnesses affecting the cardiovascular or respiratory systems.

Anxiety and agitation:

People with dyspnea may suffer anxiety and restlessness because their breathing becomes difficult.

It's vital to note that dyspnea is a symptom, not a particular diagnosis. Determining the primary reason behind dyspnea is key for effective treatment. People who have severe or chronic dyspnea should receive medical care right once for a full assessment and diagnosis.

CHAPTER TWO

Recognition

In order to discover the underlying reason of the complaint, a thorough medical evaluation is necessary for the diagnosis of dyspnea, or shortness of breath. The following aspects could be a part of the diagnostic process:

Background Information on Health:

A detailed medical history that includes information on the onset, course, and aspects of the dyspnea will be collected by the healthcare expert. They will ask about any triggering factors, related symptoms, and the existence of any underlying medical conditions.

Physical Evaluation:

There will be a full physical examination to determine cardiovascular and pulmonary health.

This could comprise monitoring for respiratory distress, watching chest movement, monitoring heart rate and rhythm, and listening to lung sounds.

Diagnostic Examinations:

Depending on the probable underlying cause of the dyspnea, a number of diagnostic tests may be prescribed. These examinations could consist of:

PFTs, or pulmonary function tests, examine the capacity and function of the lungs.

A chest X-ray or CT scan can be performed to picture the chest and discover any irregularities in the heart, lungs, or chest wall.

Blood tests: Look for disorders such electrolyte imbalances, infections, and anemia.

Electrocardiogram, generally known as an EKG or ECG: Capture the heart's electrical activity to discover irregularities.

Echocardiogram: Use ultrasonography to analyze the heart's composition and operation.

Measure the levels of carbon dioxide and oxygen in arterial blood with the Arterial Blood Gas (ABG) Test.

Exercise Stress Test: Assess respiratory and cardiovascular capability when engaging in physical exercise.

Spirometry: Determine how much and how rapidly you can breathe in and out.

Imaging of the chest:

X-rays and CT scans are types of chest imaging that can be used to discover infections, fluid buildup in the lungs, and structural issues.

Heart Examination:

Tests such as echocardiography, stress tests, or cardiac catheterization may be used to examine cardiac function in order to monitor blood flow and highlight heart-related disorders.

Professional Guidance:

The medical professional may recommend the patient for extra assessment to pulmonologists, cardiologists, or other suitable specialists based on the results.

Observing:

In certain instances, continued monitoring—such as ambulatory Holter monitoring for irregular heart rhythms or nocturnal oximetry for assessments of oxygen levels during sleep—may be indicated.

Evaluation of Mental Health:

If dyspnea is caused by psychological or anxiety-related disorders, a mental health evaluation might be carried out.

The individual's symptoms, medical history, and physical examination results are taken into consideration when creating the diagnostic strategy. The underlying cause of dyspnea can be addressed with the correct management and treatment options once a diagnosis has been made. For a full examination, those who suffer severe or chronic dyspnea must obtain medical care as soon as feasible.

Treatment Options

The underlying cause of dyspnea, or shortness of breath, must be discovered by a full medical evaluation in order to guide treatment. The purpose of management strategies is to treat the individual ailment that is generating dyspnea. Based on prevalent causes, the following broad therapeutic techniques are suggested:

Conditions Related to the Respiratory System:

Inhaled corticosteroids and bronchodilators are examples of anti-inflammatory medications that may be used for asthma. Controller drugs are a viable aspect of long-term management strategies.

Inhaled corticosteroids, oxygen therapy, and bronchodilators may be recommended for Chronic Obstructive Pulmonary Disease (COPD). Programs for pulmonary rehabilitation can promote general health and respiratory function.

Heart Failure:

Pharmaceuticals such as angiotensin receptor blockers (ARBs), ACE inhibitors, beta-blockers, and diuretics may be suggested to treat the symptoms of heart failure and enhance cardiac function.

It may be advised to undertake lifestyle improvements, such as dietary adjustments and fluid restriction.

Heart Hypertension:

It may be required to prescribe some therapies for pulmonary hypertension or drugs like vasodilators.

Infections

To treat respiratory infections, doctors may prescribe antibiotics or antiviral medicines.

Anemia

It may be advised to take iron supplements or undertake other therapies that deal with the underlying cause of anemia.

Overweight:

It may be recommended to regulate weight through food and exercise in order to treat obesity-related dyspnea.

Panic or Anxiety Disorders:

Treatment options may include anti-anxiety medicines, relaxation strategies, and cognitive-behavioral therapy (CBT).

GERD, or gastroesophageal reflux disease:

Adjusting one's diet and sleeping posture to elevate the head can be two lifestyle decisions that can help manage dyspnea associated with GERD. Drugs that reduce the formation of acid may also be advised.

Environmental Factors:

It could be advised to stay away from allergens or toxins in the surroundings. Supplemental oxygen or respiratory support may be required in certain instances.

Neuromuscular Conditions:

It may be thought about addressing underlying neuromuscular issues and giving non-invasive ventilation for breathing aid.

Modification of Medication:

If a medicine is causing dyspnea as a side effect, it might be necessary to adjust it under a doctor's supervision.

Physical Therapy:

Programs for pulmonary rehabilitation and exercise can be helpful for patients whose dyspnea is caused by deconditioning or inactivity.

Dyspnea sufferers must engage closely with medical professionals to discover the best course of action for their individual dyspnea scenario. To treat the intricacy of the underlying reasons, a multidisciplinary strategy involving cardiologists, pulmonologists, and other professionals may be required in some cases. The critical parts of an effective dyspnea treatment strategy are early intervention and continued care.

Handling Severe Dyspnea

Acute dyspnea, which is defined by a quick and severe onset of dyspnea, must be addressed with immediate assessment and intervention to treat the underlying cause. The general steps for addressing abrupt dyspnea are as follows:

Immediate Medical Attention:

It is vital to receive emergency medical care right once if someone is having acute dyspnea, particularly if it is severe or accompanied by chest tightness, confusion, or cyanosis (bluish staining). Visit the closest emergency department or give the emergency services a call.

First Evaluation:

During the initial examination, medical personnel will look at the patient's overall clinical state, oxygen saturation levels, and vital signs (heart rate, blood pressure, and respiration rate).

Treatment utilizing Oxygen:

To raise the blood's oxygen levels, extra oxygen may be supplied. A face mask, nasal cannula, or non-invasive ventilation may be employed, depending on the patient's response and the degree of dyspnea.

Orientation:

It could be useful to arrange the patient such that breathing is easier. Leaning forward or sitting upright, for instance, can enhance respiratory mechanics and reduce breathing difficulties.

Administration of Medication:

Medication may be used for acute dyspnea, depending on what triggered it. This could include diuretics for heart failure, bronchodilators for diseases like COPD or asthma, or medications to treat other special causes.

Fluids injected intravenously:

Intravenous fluids may be given sometimes to alleviate dehydration or boost heart function.

Observation and Diagnostic Examinations:

It is necessary to regularly assess cardiac rhythm, oxygen saturation, and vital signs. To determine the underlying cause, diagnostic procedures like electrocardiograms (ECGs), blood tests, and chest X-rays may be conducted.

Addressing the Root Cause:

Targeted treatment actions are started as soon as the root problem is recognized. Depending on the diagnosis, certain drugs, therapies, or procedures can be required.

Assistive Healthcare:

It may be possible to incorporate supportive care strategies including pain management, anxiety treatment, and emotional support into the management strategy.

Advisory of Experts:

Sometimes, experts with specific knowledge in treating the illness causing acute dyspnea, including cardiologists or pulmonologists, are contacted.

Admission to Hospital:

A hospital admission may be required for additional monitoring, treatment, and evaluation of acute dyspnea, depending on its severity and underlying cause.

The underlying cause must be taken into consideration when managing acute dyspnea. Optimizing results requires early and accurate diagnosis in addition to timely start of relevant therapies. People who have acute dyspnea should get in touch with a doctor right away so they can be properly assessed and treated quickly.

Coping Mechanisms and Assistance

Dyspnea requires self-management techniques, lifestyle modifications, and asking for help from friends, family, and medical specialists. For those who are suffering dyspnea, the following coping mechanisms and supportive actions might be used:

Observe Medical Advice

Follow the advice and treatment plan that the medical staff has prescribed. Respect prescription drug instructions and show up for follow-up visits.

Acquire and Apply Breathing Methods:

Breathing techniques like diaphragmatic breathing and pursed lips breathing can help control dyspnea and enhance respiratory health. The goal of these methods is to improve oxygen exchange by breathing slowly and deliberately.

Exercises for Pacing:

Divide work and activities into more manageable chunks, and take pauses as necessary. To save energy, pace yourself and refrain from overdoing it.

CHAPTER THREE

Orientation:

Look for positions that are comfortable and help with breathing. Breathing problems can often be alleviated for many by sitting up straight or elevating the upper body with more pillows.

Fan or airflow usage:

Air circulation can be improved and comfort levels raised by placing fans to provide a light breeze or by utilizing the airflow from an open window.

Retain Hydration:

Staying well hydrated promotes respiratory and general health. It's crucial to speak with medical professionals because some people need to adhere to particular hydration limitations.

Observe Environmental Stressors:

Recognize and stay away from environmental irritants like smoke, allergies, or pollution that might exacerbate dyspnea.

Managing Body Weight:

If appropriate, focus on eating a balanced diet and getting regular exercise to help you reach and stay at a healthy weight. Controlling weight can improve cardiovascular and respiratory health.

Practice Calming Techniques:

Reduced stress and anxiety can help prevent dyspnea, as can mindfulness, meditation, and guided imagery.

Get Emotional Assistance:

Discuss your thoughts and feelings with dependable family members, friends, or support networks. During trying circumstances, emotional support can offer consolation and understanding.

Exercise and Recovery:

Engage in organized physical rehabilitation programs, particularly if dyspnea is associated with chronic illnesses such as COPD or deconditioning. These initiatives emphasize physical activity, education, and enhancing general wellbeing.

Modifications to the Home:

Make changes to the living space to lessen physical strain. To make a space more accessible, think about adding handrails, utilizing assistive technology, or moving furniture around.

Make a Plan:

Arrange events and trips ahead of time, taking into account things like accessibility, seats that are available, and possible triggers. Making a plan can help you feel more prepared and less anxious.

Remain Up to Date:

Learn as much as you can about the choices for treating your particular ailment. Being informed enables patients to take an active role in their care and interact with medical professionals in an efficient manner.

Support Teams:

Joining online forums or support groups can give you a place to meet people going through similar things, talk about your experiences, and trade coping mechanisms.

Keep in mind that every person's experience with dyspnea is different, and experimenting to find individualized coping mechanisms may be necessary. The management plan will be in line with each patient's needs and objectives if there is open communication with healthcare practitioners.

The underlying cause, treatment efficacy, and general health of the patient all influence the prognosis and long-term management of dyspnea. Taking into account prognosis and long-term care are the following:

Determining the Root Cause and Addressing It:

The precise diagnosis and treatment of the particular ailment producing dyspnea frequently determine the prognosis. Providing adequate care for cardiovascular or respiratory disorders might greatly enhance the results in the long run.

Chronic Illnesses:

People who have long-term respiratory disorders such as COPD or asthma may go through periods of stability and flare-ups. Adherence to recommended medication regimens, lifestyle adjustments, and routine follow-up visits with healthcare experts are all part of long-term therapy.

Heart Conditions:

Long-term treatment for dyspnea associated with cardiovascular diseases, such as heart failure or coronary artery disease, involves taking drugs to control symptoms and enhance heart function. For general cardiovascular health, lifestyle modifications including frequent exercise and a heart-healthy diet are essential.

Respiratory Rehabilitation:

Programs for pulmonary rehabilitation may be very important for the long-term treatment of dyspnea. These initiatives emphasize physical activity, instruction, and community building to enhance respiratory health and general well-being.

Management of Medication:

Taking prescription drugs as directed is crucial to controlling dyspnea brought on by long-term illnesses. Depending on the underlying cause, this may involve bronchodilators, diuretics, anti-inflammatory drugs, or other treatments.

Modifications to Lifestyle:

Long-term care requires a healthy lifestyle that is adopted and maintained. This include controlling stress, abstaining from tobacco use, eating a balanced diet, and exercising to the best of one's abilities.

Frequent observation and follow-up:

Cardiovascular and respiratory health can be continuously monitored with routine check-ups with medical professionals. Treatment regimens may need to be modified in response to evolving symptoms, test findings, or general health conditions.

Treatment utilizing Oxygen:

Improved oxygenation may benefit those needing long-term oxygen therapy for chronic respiratory disorders, improving their quality of life. Adherence to the recommended oxygen concentrations is essential for efficiency.

Instructions for Patients:

Acquiring knowledge about the illness, available therapies, and self-care techniques enables people to take an active role in their own care. Long-term wellbeing depends on knowing when to seek medical assistance and recognizing the warning signals of exacerbations.

Support for Mental Health:

For long-term wellbeing, dyspnea's emotional effects must be managed. Counseling or therapy as well as other mental health services can assist people manage the anxiety or despair brought on by long-term respiratory or cardiovascular diseases.

Planning for Advanced Care:

Advanced care planning and end-of-life preferences should be discussed with loved ones and healthcare providers for those with advanced or progressive diseases.

It is noteworthy that the long-term management of dyspnea is customized according to the individual's overall health, co-existing diseases, and the specific diagnosis. Improved prognosis and long-term well-being are facilitated by proactive self-management, regular communication with healthcare practitioners, and a holistic approach to health.

CONCLUSION

In summary, dyspnea, often known as shortness of breath, is a complicated symptom that may result from a number of cardiovascular, respiratory, or other medical issues. It can have a profound effect on a person's everyday activities, emotional health, and general quality of life. In order to treat dyspnea, a comprehensive medical examination is necessary to determine the underlying cause. Targeted therapies and long-term strategies are then employed.

The successful diagnosis and treatment of the particular ailment causing the symptom will determine the prognosis for those suffering with dyspnea. Improving results and long-term well-being are mostly dependent on early diagnosis, following treatment regimens, and making lifestyle changes.

The key to managing dyspnea is coping mechanisms such breathing exercises, lifestyle modifications, and emotional support. A more proactive and empowered strategy to managing dyspnea involves participating in pulmonary rehabilitation, remaining aware about the underlying illness, and keeping constant touch with healthcare experts.

Even though dyspnea can present difficulties, prospects for a better quality of life and optimism are provided by ongoing research, advances in medical care, and a multidisciplinary approach to therapy. Getting prompt medical attention, adhering to recommended treatment regimens, and embracing a holistic perspective on health are essential components in managing the intricacies of dyspnea and enhancing general wellbeing.

In order to improve their health and handle the unique difficulties brought on by shortness of breath, people with dyspnea are urged to actively engage in self-management techniques, collaborate with medical professionals, and be a member of support networks.

THE END